Table of Contents:

Disclaimers

Background

Benefits

Preparation

Exercise

Diet

Fasting

Motivations

Maintaining

Speeding Up Weight Loss

Blood Tests Comparison (Pre/Post Diet)

Summary

1. DISCLAIMERS

- The author is not a physician, nor do I claim to be a weight management expert. Please consult your physician before starting this or any diet or exercise routine.
- You are not allowed to reprint or resell this book without express written permission from the author.
- The author makes no claims of how much weight you can lose with this method, as each person's metabolism is different, but I was able to lose 40lbs in six months. Since everyone comes in different sizes and has different metabolic rates, you may lose less or more weight than I did, but you will lose weight if you follow these simple steps to dieting and exercising.
- The author is not responsible for a person using the diet and exercises in this book.
- By reading this document, the reader agrees that under no circumstances is the author responsible for any losses, direct or indirect, which incur as a result of the use of information contained within this document, including, but not limited to, errors, omissions, or inaccuracies.
- The purchases of recommended products using the links within this book may earn the author a referral fee. The author only recommends products that assisted him in this diet.
- Copyright © 2020 by John Zur
  - All rights reserved. No part of this book may be reproduced in any manner without the express written consent of the author, except in the case of

brief excerpts in critical reviews or articles.

2. BACKGROUND

Up until my late forties, I was considered thin or "flaco," as my Spanish friend's family used to call me (meaning "skinny").
I was the kind of guy who could eat anything and never gain weight. I averaged about five pints of ice cream a week since I was about thirteen!

I was the type of guy who couldn't understand why other people had weight problems. I would think that they must be lazy or lack discipline.

Although I worked long hours and did a lot of traveling, I had a high metabolic rate, and I enjoyed playing sports, running, or just shooting baskets until the night fell.

Then in my late forties I was doing a bench press in my basement, with no one around but my dog, when I decided to go for one more rep. I couldn't get it up to the bar holder. I was in a narrow section of my basement and couldn't roll the bar and weights off me. So, I did something stupid ... given my options, I didn't have much choice since I didn't think my dog was going to help. I arched my back and pushed the weight back up to the holder.

That was the start of severe back problems. Sports and exercise were out of the question for months. Given my age, my metabolism was also slowing down. In a year's time, I had gained at least 60lbs. I struggled with these pounds until this past year—a twelve-year period!

I gained empathy and respect for all those people who weren't as lucky as myself during my first forty-eight years, and had been battling their weight gain. How naive I had been.

I was tired of wearing Hawaiian shirts to disguise my gut. In reality, they boldly and loudly announced: *"Look at me, I have a big gut, but you're all going to be fooled by my Hawaiian shirt!"*

I tried those elastic t-shirts and Velcro stomach wraps that were supposed to make me look slimmer when all they did was cause me to sweat profusely and gag for air.

Due to my poor self-image, I made up excuses not to see friends and family nor go out in public much. In the process, I missed a lot of wonderful and cherished moments that I'll never get back. Plus, my friends and family thought I was "dissing" them and weren't too happy with me missing so many functions.

I used to do a one-mile walk around my neighborhood—mostly walking my dog or just enjoying a nice evening. The extra weight caused my legs to cramp and gave me shin splints. I would literally have to walk up the last hill to my home backwards to use different leg muscles. Otherwise I'd have to sit on the curb for twenty minutes to recuperate.

One particularly embarrassing time was when I organized a work reunion Christmas party. Many of the people attending had to ask some of my friends who I was!

One of the final straws was when I volunteered for a Community Art Theater as an usher. I was on my way to the orientation and had to park three blocks away. Even though it wasn't that hot, by the time I'd walked two blocks, I was out of breath and soaked with sweat. I was so embarrassed that I turned around and went home. I not only lost the rewarding opportunity of volunteer work, I let the theater down because they had to hustle to find a replacement.

After twelve years of weight gain and loss, up and down, I

finally decided to come up with a strategy to lose 40lbs. I wanted to get to a healthy weight, where I could wear "normal" clothes and not worry about a gut. Over those past twelve years I'd found swimming as a way to build up my upper body muscle. Now, I just needed to get rid of the weight in my belly, rear, neck and face.

I decided, as an engineer, to *bypass all the fad diets that usually resulted in a person putting the weight back on within six to twelve months after the diet.*

I decided to *use common sense and discipline.* My theory was that I could eat the foods that I normally ate, but in smaller portions. Combined with exercise and fasting one day a week, I would attain my goal while also indulging in the food I love on the weekends (i.e., pasta, pizza and beer, etc.).

By not changing my diet drastically, I would be able to *maintain* my weight going forward.

I'm proud to say that this strategy worked: I successfully lost 40lbs in six months and have maintained that weight ever since.

This is the guide to that successful strategy!

Never again will you have to put avatars or old photos up on social media, you can post the REAL photo of you.

3. BENEFITS

The strategy outlined in this book can be used to lose just a few annoying pounds or many pounds. Just follow the process until you reach your goal, which could be a couple of weeks or six months (as my case in order to lose 40lbs). This helped me lose a little less than 2lbs per week. By losing only a couple of pounds a week it will be easier to maintain your weight loss in the future.

- Self confidence
- Losing 40lbs took ten years off my age!
- Enjoy pics and selfies
- Lower blood sugar
- **Lower cholesterol**
- Reduce resting heart beats per minute
    - **Heart not as stressed**
- Reduce aches and pains throughout my body
    - Less pressure on my knees and back
- Dropped three pant sizes and two shirt sizes
    - Luckily, I kept clothes from when I was thinner, but it's still enjoyable to buy new clothes!
- Easy getting in/out of car
- Increased energy level
- Increased endurance
- Increased stamina
- Biking better than twenty-five years ago
- Increased libido leading to an enhanced sex life
- Stylish clothing choices
- Mentally stronger

4. PREPARATION

1. Fitbit or Exercise Watch that tracks calories burned.
    a. Wear the Fitbit 24x7 as it also tracks your sleep and heart rate.
2. Scale.
    a. Weigh yourself once a week.
3. Spreadsheet.
    a. Use a spreadsheet or a piece a paper and pen to log your weekly weight.
    b. The Fitbit also keeps track of your weight. Make sure to log your weight loss and any other info you find valuable, at least monthly.
4. Buy yourself a good bike.
    a. A good bike is more enjoyable and motivational to ride.
    b. Same with other sports, invest in quality gear.
    c. Map out bike routes to keep things interesting, using a Bike APP. I use https://ridewithgps.com/ and I can find existing routes or create new ones. It provides GPS turn-by-turn directions. It costs less than ten bucks a month.
    d. Use a bike phone holder to follow route directions.
    e. If your hands get numb after riding a while, I recommend raising the handlebars and

getting ergonomic grips.
   f. For safety I recommend a powerful light, a solid helmet, and an attachable mirror.
5. Map out walks to keep things interesting and have different lengths depending on the weather and how much other exercise you already did.
   a. Use Google Maps.
6. Stop smoking (if applicable).
7. Buy good walking shoes or sneakers.
   a. I find New Balance the best since I have wide feet and get the extra wide width. Not many other manufacturers provide this width.
   b. I also highly recommend getting orthotics for better support and cushioning when going for longer walks.
8. Discipline: Prepare yourself mentally for a six-month project.
9. Get a physical with complete blood work prior to starting this diet. After you attain your goal, get another physical and compare the blood work pre/post diet.
10. Use ice packs after exercising to reduce inflammation.
11. Wear safety accessories when walking at night: Arm Bands and Reflective Vests.
12. Use a webcam or your phone to take similarly positioned photos each week and compare all the photos after reaching your goal.
13. Join a health club, if you think it will be more helpful than exercising on your own.
   a. Many healthcare plans provide great discounts when joining a health club.
14. Get a large bag of dog food or something equivalent to your target weight loss (large dog food bags usually weigh around 40lbs).

        a. Carry that up and down the stairs a few times to get a real feel of how much extra weight you are carrying and how good you'll feel when it's off!

15.   Tell some friend and family about the goal you are trying to accomplish—this will help you to be more accountable. You don't want to let them down, but more importantly you don't want to let yourself down and this will help you to avoid excuses.

Note 1: If you cannot afford to purchase a Fitbit, or join a gym, or buy a new bicycle, that's no problem; walking is free! Just use the tools available to you and keep track of your weight on a weekly basis to see how you are progressing towards your goal.

Note 2: Some of the links above may not work on apple devices, if that is the case, please copy and paste the links below into your browser.

Fitbit: https://amzn.to/2G9Mn0c
Scale: https://amzn.to/36m5q26
Bike Phone Holder: https://amzn.to/33cpEcL
Handlebars: https://amzn.to/3ih4deW
Ergonomic Grips: https://amzn.to/33e41Zn
Powerful Light: https://amzn.to/3cJmb8B
Solid Helmet: https://amzn.to/349XEpx
Attachable Mirror: https://amzn.to/2Sdqxvc
Sneakers: https://amzn.to/3jgZzPm
Orthotics: https://amzn.to/3cGLybj
Ice Packs: https://amzn.to/2GjrOOH
Arm Bands: https://amzn.to/36fertT
Reflective Vests: https://amzn.to/345mdnq

5. EXERCISE

My main focus in exercising was to burn calories. My goal each day was to burn 2500 calories. Over time, I also lowered my resting heart rate BPM (Beats Per Minute) from 80BPM to 62BPM.

Follow my exact exercise routine or choose your own, but always aim to burn a similar number of calories per day and to reduce your resting heart BPM.

Use your Fitbit or other device to measure burned calories, and focus on doing the types of exercises you enjoy. For me, it was biking, walking, and some golfing.

Always warm up and stretch before doing any exercises, and drink plenty of water prior to and after exercising.

Typical: 45-90 minutes of activity

Great exercises:

- Biking
    - Push yourself to bike the hill versus walking the bike
    - Follow different routes to keep things interesting
    - Select routes at all levels of difficulty
- Walking
    - Bring the dog along
    - Drive to scenic parks or a quiet area for walks with a partner or alone
    - Listen to music or podcasts while walking
- Swimming

- House and yard work
- Golfing
    - No carts when golfing—walk
- Sex
- Limited weight lifting
- Use stairs instead of elevators
- Badminton
- Tennis
- Ping Pong you'd be surprised at the calories you will burn
- Walk or bike to store vs driving
- Use the Fitbit reminder to meet hourly steps and to get up from the couch or desk to walk around a bit

*Don't miss a day, even if it's just walking the dog a short distance
*Stay Hydrated
*Use safety when exercising
*Change-up exercises, routes, and/or pace when you hit a plateau

Post Exercise:

- Stretch
- Ibuprofen or Tylenol and ice
- Foot massager
- Body massages as reward after every 5lbs lost

6. DIET

Follow my exact diet or choose similar foods with similar the same amount calories, carbs, and sugars. My eating goal was to eat mostly healthy foods in smaller portions and simply burn more calories than I was taking in on a daily basis.

- Eat low carbs and low sugar. Choose proteins and small portions (appetizer portion or 50% of normal entrée).
- Avoid deep-fried foods.
- Still enjoy food and drink, but spread them out in smaller portions.
  - It will enable you to maintain the weight loss since you are basically eating the same foods and not doing an extreme diet.
- Alcohol and fun meals on Fridays or Saturdays.

Weekday Food:

Breakfast:
- Post Honey Bunches of Oats w/Almonds
- Kashi GoLean Crunch—Honey and Almond
- Soy milk
- One slice of Ezekiel Bread with guacamole
- Chobani Yogurt (Key Lime)

Lunch: SKIP

Dinner:
- Fish (steamed or grilled)—lightly seasoned (no heavy sauces or marinades, and eat the skin).
  - Rainbow trout

- - Salmon
  - Cod
- Steak (grilled)—salt and pepper
  - Skirt steak
  - Rib-Eye
- Slices of ham
- Burgers without buns
- Chicken (dark meat without skin)
- Falafel & couscous
- Soups.
  - Lentils
  - Chicken and rice
- Salads.
  - Spinach or red leaf lettuce
  - Tomatoes
  - Cucumbers
  - Light dressing (fat-free raspberry vinaigrette)
- Sweet potatoes
- Veggies
  - Brussels sprout (grilled or steamed)
  - Broccoli
  - Cauliflower
  - String beans
  - Fresh corn
  - Le Sueur sweet peas
- Tall glass of Metamucil (amazing how this will fill you up and it's great for bowel movements)
- Brown and/or wild rice
- Chicken breast or tuna with light Mayo on Ezekiel Bread, or by itself

Snacks:
- Almonds
- Raisins
- Pickles
- 100 calorie microwave popcorn

- Sliced honey golden crisp apple
- Fruit as snack—satisfies sweet tooth
- Small pieces of cut-up ham

Beverages:
- Water
- Dell lemonade after a workout
- Metamucil with water

Weekend Food:

Breakfast:
- Eggs and sausages
- One slice of Ezekiel Bread with guacamole and a sunny side egg

Lunch: SKIP

Dinner:
- Pasta (average portion) with tomato sauce
- Pizza (two or three slices)
- Chicken fingers
- Perogies
- Sushi
- Burger on bun
- Eggplant or chicken parmigiana

Snacks:
- Two or three cookies
- Small bag of chips or popcorn
- Fruit as snack—satisfies sweet tooth

Beverages: (one of below)
- Beer four to six bottles
- Wine two to three glasses
- Champagne two to three glasses

7. FASTING

Please check with your doctor before including fasting in your diet.

Twenty-four-hour fast one day a week (Mon–Thurs).
Stay occupied on fast days: read, PC work, games, TV binge, long walk, etc. (The day will go by faster)
Drink plenty of water

8. MOTIVATIONS

- Motivations to start:
  - No more avoiding friends and family
  - Avoiding a nursing home
  - Improved confidence
  - Not having to walk backwards
  - Not having difficulty with getting out of a chair, off a couch, and out of the car
  - Less knee, foot, and joint pain
  - Lower cholesterol
  - Stronger heart
  - Better quality of life
- Motivations to continue:
  - If you're tired and sore—don't stop! You will feel a sense of achievement versus disappointment
    - Unless you feel that the pain is not just from soreness, then see your doctor
  - It's great to have a partner or friend/family cheer you on, or work out with you
  - You will love the way you feel so much that you won't want to destroy everything you've worked for.
  - Don't be frustrated when two or three weeks go by without weight loss
    - Your body is adjusting to a new routine
    - It can simply be a time to switch things up
    - Weight loss will begin again within a week or two
  - Reward intermediate goals

- Don't get frustrated, you are doing something very difficult
- Your momentum and drive will kick in when pounds start to shred
- Identify yourself as a healthy person and continue to ask yourself what would a healthy person do regarding eating and exercise or in avoiding certain bad habits – THINK LIKE A HEALTHY PERSON

9. MAINTAINING

I still fast one day a week, but now eat whatever I want on Fridays and Saturdays (without overindulging) and drink my alcohol or mixed drinks.

At first you might be upset to see your stomach bloated from the food and drink the next morning, but by maintaining this healthy diet and exercise, and fasting one day within the Sunday through Thursday timeframe, you *will* stay fit and healthy.

It's not about a defined weight-loss but rather identifying as a healthy person (a change in your mindset) and continuing to use this process and strategy to lose and then maintain your weight.

Stop chasing numbers after the ultimate goal.
Use a mirror, notice how clothes fit and how you feel.
THINK LIKE A HEALTHY PERSON!

10. SPEEDING UP WEIGHT LOSS

Note that this will make maintaining your weight loss more difficult after achieving your goal, and it's not an option for everyone. But ... if you want to speed up your weight loss, go into full-on boot-camp mode by using the weekday diet all seven days of the week.

11. AUTHOR'S BLOOD TESTS COMPARISON (PRE/POST DIET)

3/4/2020	8/25/2020	Comments
Hemoglobin A1c 4.5-5.7 5.6	Hemoglobin A1c 4.8-5.6 5.5	Prediabetes: 5.7 - 6.4 Diabetes: >6.4 Glycemic control for adults with diabetes: <7.0
Glucose 70-99 101	Glucose 65-99 91	Lower Blood Sugar Level
Cholesterol <200 170 Triglycerides <150 235 HDL Cholesterol 46-120 29 LDL Cholesterol <100 94 Cholesterol/HDL	Cholesterol, Total 100-199 170 Triglycerides 0-149 147 HDL Cholesterol >39 41 LDL Cholesterol Calc 0-99 92 VLDL Cholesterol Cal	Reduction in most Cholesterol levels

3.4-5.0 5.9 **LDL/HDL Ratio** **0.0-3.2** **3.2** **Pulse Rate 76 /min**	5-40 31 **LDL/HDL Ratio** **0.0-3.6** **2.6** **Pulse Rate 64 /min**

12. SUMMARY

Thank you for reading this book.

Remember, following the strategy outlined helped me lose 40lbs in under six months. It works. You *will* need discipline, but once you start to see the weight dropping, it will inspire you to continue. You might hit plateaus where you exercised more than the previous week and ate less, but your weight went up. This will happen as your body gets used to the changes in your diet and exercise. This is when you need to follow the tips under "Motivation," and to mix up your exercises, routes, and pace, as well as your diet. Try not to get frustrated. Within a week or two, the weight will begin dropping again.

Whenever you find yourself retreating back to the old unhealthy lifestyle, refer back to this book. It will get you back on the path to success.

Should you find success by following the strategy outlined in this book, please rate my book on Amazon and provide a written review. I will be extremely grateful.

https://amzn.to/35GXlnR
(If link doesn't work, please copy and paste into your browser)

I believe this book will help you attain your weight loss goals as it did for myself. I want to thank Tami Zorge, Brandon Zenner, Barbara Willis, Kate Zalusky, Matt Duval and Patricia Zur for their help in editing and reviewing this book along with Cheryl Kaye Tardif for her great insights into marketing and publishing an e-book and my very understanding and supportive fiancé, Christine Yang, for always being there for me.

BACK COVER

"A no-nonsense diet guide from a regular guy whose common-sense approach to weight loss is both relatable and not intimidating. This just may be the book that helps shed those stubborn pounds once and for all."

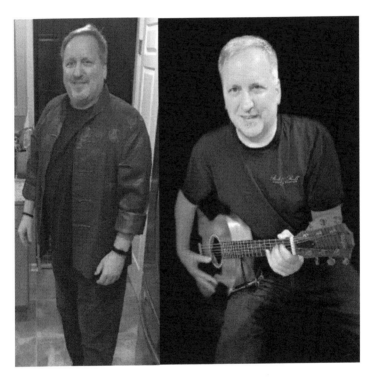

Before and After Photos of the Author

Contact the Author at: MakeMeTHINAgainPlease@gmail.com
Or Visit the Author's Facebook page at:
https://www.facebook.com/Make-Me-THIN-Again-112829053967508/?modal=admin_todo_tour

Made in the USA
Columbia, SC
27 September 2022

68032498R00015